This Book Belongs To

Printed in Great Britain
by Amazon

55301654R00070